Table of Contents

Introduction

What is multiple sclerosis?

Multiple sclerosis also known as MS is a disease that affects the central nervous system, ranging from the brain to the spinal cord as well as the optic nerve in the eye. This causes problems to muscle control, balance, vision as well as other body functions.

The most complicated side of this disease is that it is different for everyone who has this disease with each of them, having different effects. Some individuals, when affected with multiple sclerosis, have trouble with any of their daily activities, needing treatment in the end. While others, have mild symptoms and don't require any treatment whatsoever.

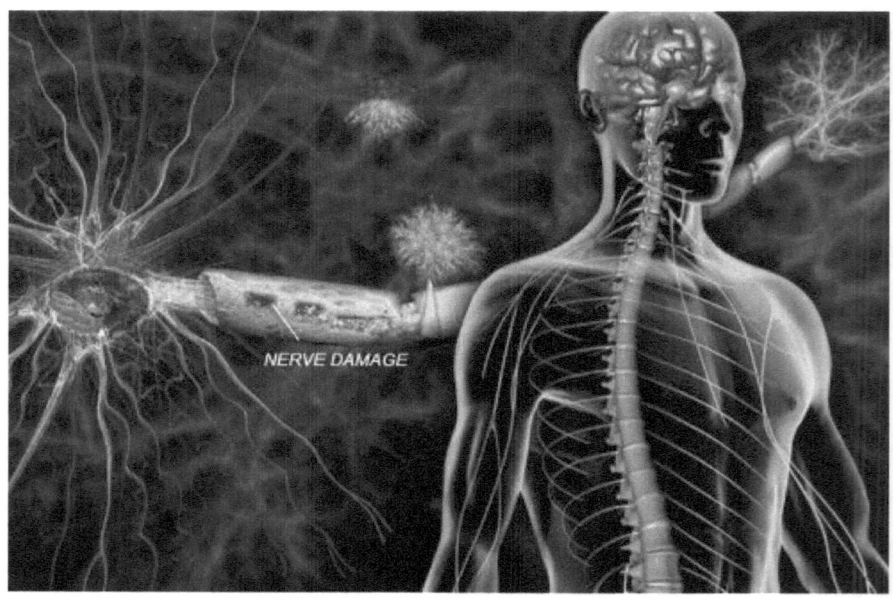

NERVE DAMAGE

Multiple sclerosis occurs when your immune system attacks a fatty material in the body known as myelin, which covers the nerve fiber to protect them. This cover is lost after the attack leaving the nerve open and eventually damaged with the result being the formation of scar tissues.

At the end of all this, the brain cannot send signals through the body properly with the nerves malfunctioning leaving your movement and sense of feeling impeded.

As a result of this, you may have symptoms like:

- Sexual problems
- Trouble walking
- Blurred or double vision
- Numbness and tingling
- Poor bowel or bladder control
- Problems remembering or focusing
- Pain
- Depression
- Feeling tired
- Muscle spasms or weakness

Most of these symptoms start between the ages of 20 to 30 with of them coming as attacks especially when the condition becomes worse. When these symptoms improve over time for those who experience improvements, things get better, and for some, it only gets worse.

Scientists have found many treatments for multiple sclerosis to help prevent these attacks, as well as slow down the effect of this disease.

Causes of Multiple Sclerosis

This part of the subject is somewhat a controversial one as at yet because the cause of multiple sclerosis is one of much controversy. However, we know a couple of things that would make the disease unlikely.

Some people contact multiple sclerosis after a viral infection which disturbs the normal functionality of the immune system, as well as triggering the disease in the process.

Others contact multiple sclerosis via smoking while for some, they stand a higher chance of contacting the disease due to their gene type. The point is that compared to other diseases which we can rightfully point to the cause of the disease, all we have is a hypothesis.

Possible causes of Multiple sclerosis

With the existence of uncertainties concerning the major causes of multiple sclerosis, we look at some of the possible reasons.

Malfunctioning immune system

We all know that Multiple sclerosis is an autoimmune condition, one which is in a particular sense, very humorous. Why is that? Well, something signals your immune system to attack the body with the point of attack being the myelin, a fatty substance which covers the nerve fiber in the central nervous system (the brain and spinal cord). The Myelin protects the nerves, sort of like the plastic that protects your charger and when it is messed up, it leaves your nerves in a position where it can not send messages the way they usually would. Meaning it is open to damages as well as other infections.

Contacting other autoimmune diseases like diabetes, inflammatory bowel disease, and thyroid can also leave you open to contacting multiple sclerosis.

Environmental factors
People of certain ethnic groups, as well as individuals who live in certain places of the world notably cooler places like northern Europe, are more likely to contact Multiple sclerosis. If you move to a place where multiple sclerosis is common as a teenager, your chances of contacting multiple sclerosis become high. The reason why cold environments seem to be a factor is as a result of the amount of sunlight taken in. In most of northern Europe as well as places close to the equator, there is less sunlight leaving the production of Vitamin D from sunlight very low. The lack of Vitamin D leaves

your immune system vulnerable to immune-related diseases like this one.

Smokers, as well as people who stay in an environment where they smoke often, are also prone to multiple sclerosis with their case progressing faster than that of non-smokers. Smoking leads to a clinically isolated syndrome which is the first instance of Multiple sclerosis, lasts for 24 hours and puts you in pole position for a second episode and Multiple sclerosis. (Smoking is just one of many possible triggers, it does NOT cause M.S)

Types of Multiple sclerosis

Nerve damage is a significant factor when it comes to multiple sclerosis, and although it affects a certain part of the body, each person with this disease lives with this disease in a unique way. Doctors have identified different types of Multiple Sclerosis which is a vital part of predicting how severe the condition is as well as how the treatment works.

Relapsing-Remitting Multiple Sclerosis
This counts for the majority of people with multiple sclerosis as about 84% of the population of people with this disease have this type. People in this group have their first signs in their early 20's, and after that, they have relapses from time to time, followed by a time of recovery, depending on the individual.

Most individuals with relapsing and remitting Multiple Sclerosis would move to a secondary and more progressive stage of Multiple Sclerosis.

Primary Progressive Multiple Sclerosis
At this stage of this disease, we find things gradually getting worse over time. The symptoms are not well-defined attacks, and there is hardly any point of recovery. Also, treatments that work for other forms of this disease seem not to work for this one. This form of Multiple Sclerosis accounts for 10% of the total population of the people with this disease.

We talked about the fact that this form of Multiple sclerosis is different from others and here are some ways:

- This form of Multiple sclerosis usually leads to disability earlier than the other forms.
- Individuals with primary progressive Multiple Sclerosis are at an average age of 40 showing that they are usually older when they are diagnosed.
- Compared to other forms of Multiple sclerosis where women outnumber men 3 to 1, a roughly equal number of men and women experience this form of multiple sclerosis.

Secondary Progressive Multiple Sclerosis

After going through the relapsing and remitting stage of Multiple Sclerosis, most people get secondary progressive Multiple Sclerosis. Compared to other forms of this disease where there are relapses and remissions, the symptoms come forth without on a steady note without the ease of relapsing and remission as with other types. This change happens after 10 to 15 years of being diagnosed with relapsing-remitting Multiple sclerosis.

Scientists are still unsure why the disease makes the shift, but there are a few things known about the process:

- People who are older before getting diagnosed first diagnosed have a shorter time before the disease becomes secondary progressive,
- People who find it difficult to fully recover from relapses transition faster to the Secondary Progressive Multiple Sclerosis more quickly than those who recover.
- Compared to other forms of Multiple Sclerosis, the transformation leads to a slower decline in the proper functionality of the nerves as well as a change in the process of ongoing nerve damage.

This form of Multiple Sclerosis is hard to handle as the day goes by and is generally tough to treat. The symptoms worsen at different rates depending on the person, and when it comes to treatment, it works moderately well, but people find it challenging to use their body like they used to before getting the disease.

Signs and symptoms of Multiple Sclerosis

Individuals with Multiple Sclerosis have their first Symptoms between the ages of 20-40 years of age. These symptoms for some get better and eventually start again at a later time while for some others they stay and linger around for an extended period.

Although not impossible, it is difficult to find two individuals with the same symptoms. One might be alike, but it's hard to find two people with symptoms. One might have just one symptom and go for a long time even years without having any other one. For some others, the symptoms get worse within weeks or months depending on the individual.

Keeping tabs on what's happening to you and your body is the right thing to do as it would not only help you but also your doctor on a pathway to understanding you as well as how well your treatment is going.

Here are some early signs of Multiple Sclerosis:

As we highlighted earlier in previous sections, most individuals have **clinically isolated syndrome** first before getting diagnosed with Multiple Sclerosis. This episode of this disease lasts for about a day before transition where your immune system tells the body to attack the Myelin (the protective cover of the nerves in the spine and brain) which makes it harder for signals to travel between the brain and body.

There are two types of clinically isolated syndrome:

- Monofocal episode: One Symptom
- Multifocal episode: more than one symptom

Other common symptoms of clinically isolated syndrome include:

Numbness and Tingling

Not everyone with clinically isolated syndrome gets Multiple Sclerosis. However, the chances become higher if you have lesions in your brain due to the loss of myelin. If there are other symptoms of multiple sclerosis later, then an MRI scan would be carried out on your brain.

Numbness and tingling usually tell on the legs, and when it does, you might feel the following:

- A feeling like an electric shock when you move your neck or head which can later travel down to your spine as well as into your legs and arms.

- Tingling
- Numbness on your face

Optical neuritis

This damages the nerve that connects your eye to your brain. It usually affects one eye and rarely both. When you have optical neuritis, you might notice the following:

- Blurry vision
- Eye pains, mostly when you move it
- Colors appear dull

Many people ask, could I have multiple sclerosis?

With all this information concerning multiple sclerosis and the symptoms, maybe you've often felt weak lately, or you feel your foot tingling, and when you search for these symptoms, you find out that your symptom is one of the signs of Multiple Sclerosis.

Before you start worrying because the signs and symptoms seem similar, this might be a symptom of other health conditions making it easy to confuse other conditions for multiple sclerosis.

There is a similarity to other conditions, so how can you tell if you have multiple sclerosis? You first have to understand that the first signs for these conditions start within the ages of 20 and 30 as well as other factors such as:

Tingling and Numbness

This is a lack of feeling, particularly when you cannot feel pins and needles, which makes it one of the first signs of nerve damage from Multiple Sclerosis. This can happen on the face, legs, arms or one half of the body.

Mind you; this might also occur due to lack of blood flow due to sleeping incorrectly or not moving for a very long time before you conclude.

Dizziness

Multiple sclerosis can make you feel off-balance most of the time, especially when moving around or even standing. If you feel dizzy while resting or lying down the chances are that it is a problem with the inner ear, a side which helps control your balance. Other things like medications for seizure disorders and depression need to be taken into account as well as they can also lead to dizziness.

How Multiple Sclerosis Changes Over Time

As we have highlighted severally, Multiple sclerosis is different for everyone who has it and the symptoms it causes when it flares up differ not only between people but also throughout a person's life which makes doctors say you might have Multiple Sclerosis.

Diagnosis differ based on the symptoms each person has as well as when and how they worsen and become better as well as which body parts give you problems and your test results. Really what makes this a really problematic scenario is that there is no way to predict how conditions would change as time goes by, but the good thing is that as your doctor gets the hang of how things work with your symptoms, they can help you have a more unobstructed view of how it will affect you in the future. Here are some ways in which the disease changes in each of the types of Multiple Sclerosis:

Relapsing-Remitting Multiple Sclerosis Individuals with relapsing-remitting multiple sclerosis have major attacks as symptoms worsen, known as relapses followed by either full, partial or no recovery from these relapses. These complications change over time (several days or even weeks) as well as recovery taking almost the same amount of time with some extending to months leaving symptoms getting better. This occurs for most individuals when they are first diagnosed with Multiple Sclerosis.

Primary Progressive Multiple Sclerosis
In this type of Multiple Sclerosis, symptoms worsen gradually without any obvious form of remission or relapses. Almost 15% of the population of people with Multiple Sclerosis have this type with its prominence more with people of the ages of 40 and above.

Secondary Progressive Multiple Sclerosis
People with this sort of Multiple Sclerosis start with Relapsing-Remitting Multiple Sclerosis. Later, these symptoms stop the normal progression and begin to get worse instead and this happens typically shortly after symptoms of Multiple Sclerosis begin or a long time after, depending on the person in question.

Progressive-relapsing Multiple Sclerosis

This sort of Multiple Sclerosis is the least common form of this disease with symptoms steadily becoming worse but with fewer complications and no recovery whatsoever. People with this sort of Multiple Sclerosis are first seen to have Primary-Progressive Multiple Sclerosis.

N.B: A Multiple Sclerosis Relapse starts when the brain and spinal cord nerves get swollen and irritated. Later, those nerves lose their coating which protects them, leaving a plaque-forming around them.

Multiple Sclerosis Test and Diagnosis

This disease is a challenging one when it comes to diagnosis and testing as no special test has proven very effective mostly because many other conditions have symptoms that look like Multiple Sclerosis.

Doctors who specialize in treating this disease (neurologists) have experience with diagnosis as they would ask how you are feeling and help you understand if your symptoms mean you have Multiple Sclerosis or other problems.

What exactly do doctors look out for?

As certain symptoms and signs point to Multiple Sclerosis as well as other conditions, doctors always do the following:

- Rule out any other diagnosis
- Try to prove that the damage happened at different points in time
- Look for damages around two areas of your central nervous system (i.e., spinal cord, brain, and optic nerves)

Tools for diagnosis
Concerning tools for diagnosis, doctors ask questions about medical history as well as symptoms. They will also conduct tests to see if the brain and the spinal cord are functioning correctly.

Some of these tests include:

Blood tests: blood tests do not diagnose Multiple sclerosis but a tool that points to points substances in your blood that points to it, making it easier for doctors to rule out conditions that have similar symptoms to Multiple Sclerosis.

Spinal taps: this test which is also known to some others as Lumbar Puncture, examines the fluid in the spinal column to check for high levels of protein and other factors that point to the disease. This is an excellent way to test for Multiple Sclerosis but as with many others is not full proof.

Evoked potentials: these are electrical tests which help doctors confirm if Multiple Sclerosis has affected the part of the brain which helps you feel, see, and hear. Here, they place wires on the scalp to watch your brain patterns on a screen or get electrical pulses on your legs or hands.

MRI: This is an imaging test that allows the doctor have a close look at the brain seeing the changes that caused Multiple Sclerosis especially signs like big inflammations of the deep parts of the spinal cord and brain.

However, older individuals or people with diabetes and high blood pressure can have these kinds of symptoms, so doctors consider this alongside other symptoms like your symptoms before taking diagnosis.

N.B: An MRI result which is normal does not rule out Multiple Sclerosis, but could mean you have lesions in places the scan cannot show.

Treatment for Multiple Sclerosis

For now, there is no cure for Multiple Sclerosis but lifestyle changes and medicine which basically helps you manage the progression of the disease. Here you have to work with your doctor to help find the treatment best suited for your type of Multiple Sclerosis which also causes the fewest side-effects alongside.

Here are some of the notable treatments for proper management of Multiple Sclerosis:

Disease-Modifying Drugs

For those who have Relapsing-Remitting Multiple Sclerosis, whose conditions are not getting better, doctors would initially treat you with disease-modifying drugs because these drugs slow the progression of this disease preventing it from flaring up.

These drugs help by protecting your immune system from germs, preventing it from attacking the Myelin which surrounds the nerves. Some of these drugs come as injections under the skin which makes it sore itchy or red.

Here are some of the disease-modifying drugs:

Glatiramer (Copaxone, Glatopa): this medication is the real deal as it stops your immune system from attacking the Myelin which protects and surrounds your nerves.

Beta Interferons: these are some of the most common drugs for treating Multiple Sclerosis as they ease the severity of the flares as well as the frequency of occurrence. At the initial point of usage, they cause flu-like symptoms like fatigue, fever, and aches but fade eventually after months of usage. They lower the number of white blood cells leaving your immune system incapacitated to fight anything and open to infections. They include:

- Plegridy (peginterferon beta-1a)
- Extavia (interferon beta-1b)
- Rebif (interferon beta-1a)
- Betaseron (interferon beta-1b)
- Avonex (interferon beta-1a)

Other medications can be taken as pills. Medications such as:

Fingolimod (Gilenya): this is a tablet taken once daily. To take this, if you have not had chicken pox, then you'll need a vaccine. This medicine is known for slowing down the heart rate which makes it a necessity to be watched closely by the doctor on the first dose. This drug is also linked with a rare brain infection known as Multifocal Leukoencephalopathy also known as PML.

Common side effects of this drug are headaches, coughs, back pain, and diarrhea.

Teriflunomide (Aubagio): this is a tablet taken once a day. Once you take it, the doctors would do regular tests to check how well your liver is functioning. It is not to be taken by pregnant women.

Common side effects of this disease include nausea, diarrhea and hair loss. It carries a warning from the FDA which warns against use by pregnant women because it can lead to birth defects and liver problems.

Involuntary Muscle Twitching (Myoclonus)

What is Involuntary Muscle Twitching?

People who have multiple sclerosis may often experience a muscle spasm known as Myoclonus which is the sudden twitching or Jerking of the muscles. This can last for one episode or more but basically for a few minutes.

This sort of Involuntary muscle twitching sometimes happens to people without Multiple Sclerosis, but this is common for people in this category. There are different types of Myoclonus, some of which are:

Palatal Myoclonus: this sort of Myoclonus constitutes a tremor in the roof of your mouth with another part like the face diaphragm, and tongue also involved. These twitches come fast with as many as 100 a minute.

Action Myoclonus: this is triggered by movement. It affects parts of the body like the arm, leg, face, and even the voice.

Reticular reflex Myoclonus: this causes jerking throughout your body with triggers such as movement as well as what you hear.

Brainstem myoclonus: with this sort of Myoclonus, any sort of noise or something you see might cause a smirk. Parts of your body like the neck knees and elbows may flex.

Cortical reflex myoclonus: people who have this type of myoclonus are prone to jerk-like movement in the face and upper limbs. This is the most common type of Myoclonus.

Sleep Myoclonus: this is a muscle spasm that happens while you sleep. This basically affects your lips, fingers, toes, and eyes. It might wake you u, but that rarely happens.

Symptoms of Myoclonus
Irrespective of whatever form of clonus is affecting a person, we all agree that the movement is:

- In one part of the body or all over
- Involuntary
- Sometimes severe enough to get in the way of walking, speaking, or eating.
- Shock-like
- Sudden
- Brief
- Varied in intensity and frequency

Clinically isolated syndrome

when your nervous system is attacked by your body, it is diagnosed as Multiple Sclerosis. However, when this happens once, it is considered as Clinically Isolated Syndrome. Both conditions have the same symptoms including problems with balance and muscle weakness, but people with Muscle Sclerosis have more than one episode of symptoms.

Until recently, both conditions were termed as Multiple Sclerosis, and although Clinically Isolated syndrome develops into Multiple Sclerosis, it does not always happen.

Symptoms of Clinically Isolated Syndrome
With Clinically Isolated Syndrome happening in most or some parts of the body, here are some common ones:

- Blurred vision or other eye problems
- Problems with balance or walking
- Stiffness or muscle spasms
- Muscle weakness
- Vertigo or dizziness
- Numbness or tingling in the leg, face or arm.
- Poor memory

- Bladder, sexual, or bowel problems
- Slurred speech
- Depression or mood swings
- Fatigue
- Pain

If the symptoms last for about a day, with other conditions ruled out, you are likely to be diagnosed with clinically Isolated syndrome.

Typical Causes
With Clinically Isolated Syndrome, the body attacks the Myelin (same as Multiple Sclerosis), keeping the nerves from signaling the way it normally would which normally causes your symptoms.

There are no certain reasons why the body attacks the Myelin with many believing the cause to be a virus, but that is only a theory and not a certain cause.

However, it is certain that it affects the majority of people within the ages of 20 to 30 years.

Tips for Living with Multiple Sclerosis

When you get illnesses like the flu, you know it is simply for a time, and you would eventually get better within a short period of time. However, a long-lasting condition like Multiple Sclerosis can affect your life in so many ways.

Although it does not keep you from living a happy life, because of your ability to see things from a positive perspective, you should understand that it is just a condition and does not have to define you and the way you live.

Here are sine ways to stay positive:

Take Care of Your Mind
Taking care of your mind constitutes the following:

Getting help when due

When you find it difficult to keep up with the complications that come with this disease, reach out to someone who can help. You have to understand that talking about it helps ease the mental load on you. It also helps you better manage your multiple sclerosis as well as the resulting effects.

There are many mental health practitioners who would not only listen to you but help you draw a plan that would help you gain control of your life. If this condition is also causing you to be depressed, there are medications that would also help you lift your spirit.

Find a support group

With this setting, we find other people who are also plagued with the same condition and still finding reasons to live. With this, you learn new ways to handle your condition as well as a chance to share your feelings and questions with people who understand better which helps you feel like you're not alone in this world.

Counseling

Most people do not feel sharing their issues with outsides and would rather prefer a one-on-one setting where they can talk to a therapist with their secret safe.

Keeping a diary

With this, you can write down how you are feeling per time as this would be valuable not only to share with your doctor but would help you know how things are with you and your health. With this, you can study patterns.

Control the uncertainty

With the uncertainty that comes with Multiple Sclerosis, comes the need to take charge of your life. You have to plan your life if not, life and conditions would plan for you.

Multiple Sclerosis and Exercise

Exercising helps ease the stress of Multiple Sclerosis as well as the symptoms. However, you have to be careful about the types of workouts you perform as well as the intensity you put into it. It might be difficult, but you have to understand that nothing comes easy. There is a need to work out but it is not advisable to do too much as doing that can stress the muscles, increase pain and tress the mind. Simply put, never stress the body to the point of fatigue.

Going to your doctor before you start might lead him to suggest:

- Physical limitations for your routines
- Types of exercises that are best for you as well as those you need to avoid depending on your symptoms, overall health, and fitness levels.
- How long and strong your workouts should be
- Professionals who can help you build a good and intense exercise program

Exercises for Multiple Sclerosis

Strength training: this can be done if your physician says it's okay to use resistance bands and weights to build your muscles. This is good because the stronger you are, the easier it would be to move around properly.

Stretches: this is generally good for anyone with multiple sclerosis. As they help improve muscle stiffness and spasm. It does more than the regular stretches because you have the chance to build your strength and flexibility. This also helps you fight stress and relax properly.

Aerobics: this is an exercise that helps lift your mood and get your heartbeat up. If you have weaknesses in your legs, aerobic is very great as well as walking, biking and running.

Tips for a safe workout environment

Make it fun: choose an exercise routine that you love, and you can continue with for a long time. Yoga, water aerobics and swimming work well with people with Multiple Sclerosis.

Cool down: when you complete a particular session, take out time to let your breathing, heart rate, and body temperature get back to normal before starting another one.

Always know when to stop: if you feel any pain or any sort of sickness when you're exercising, you just have to quit. If you feel a symptom flaring up, change the routine or completely stop it. Try getting a lot of rest as well as talking to your doctor to help with finding a better way to do things.

Take it slow: start every routine with a warm up and then ease into your routine. Whatever you can do should be taken slowly and improved with time. In time, you would build up your strength and do more than the initial exercise routines.

Find a balance: if you feel you can exercise vigorously, that is great but do not work out to the point that you feel weak and unable to move properly. If after the exercise, you are unable to do anything, you have to understand that you need to access your routines. Do not push yourself; do not overdo things. Stick to your normal routine and make the best out of it.

Stay safe: avoid doing things that are hazardous areas like slippery floors and places with poor lighting. Choose activities that you would be comfortable with and not likely fall down. Work with a therapist to give you the workouts that best suit you, but as for the rest of the things that concern safety. The rest is left for you.

What do you do if you get overheated? If you are sensitive to heat, and you're working out without caution, your symptoms would show up. You can avoid overheating by doing the following:

- Be aware of your body and if you notice any new symptoms, slow down or stop till you completely cool down
- Drinking a lot of cold water
- Avoid exercising during the hottest times of the day. Leaving it till the morning time when the weather is cool.
- Swimming is a good way to cool off while working out. Just make sure the environment is safe and secure.

FAQS about Multiple Sclerosis

What Is Multiple Sclerosis?

Multiple sclerosis is an issue with the immune system known as an autoimmune disease. Rather than focusing on just microorganisms, infections, and different invaders, the immune system fights the body's very own tissues. In Multiple Sclerosis, it assaults the spinal cord and the brain.

What Causes Multiple Sclerosis?

Doctors still don't comprehend why individuals get the disease; however, genetics, an individual's environment, and perhaps even viruses may play their part.

Scientists figure Multiple Sclerosis might be a condition that parents can pass to their kids through their genes. First-, second- and third-degree relatives of individuals with the illness have a higher danger of getting it.

A few researchers figure individuals may get multiple sclerosis since they're brought into the world with genes that influence their bodies to respond to a trigger in the environment. When they're exposed to it, their immune system starts targeting their own tissues.

A few investigations likewise have proposed that numerous infections might be connected with Multiple Sclerosis. In any case, there's no reasonable confirmation of a connection up until now.

What Are the Symptoms?

The principal warning signal of Multiple Sclerosis can be dramatic – to the point that an individual doesn't see them.

The most widely recognized early side effects include:

Weakness in at least one or more limbs

- Blurred vision
- Tingling
- Numbness
- Loss of balance

Less-regular cautioning signs might be:

- Lack of coordination
- Suddenly not having the capacity to move some part of your body (paralysis)
- Problems with processing data and thinking
- Slurred speech

As the sickness gets worse, other symptoms may include heat sensitivity and changes in thinking.

Can you Catch Multiple Sclerosis from Someone Else? Can you Die from It?

Multiple Sclerosis isn't viewed as a lethal sickness. Furthermore, you can't get it from another person.

In the event that other individuals in your family have the disease, you might be bound to get it sooner or later.

Is There a Cure?

No, yet there are numerous medications that can prevent the disease from worsening for some time. Alongside drugs, different treatments like physical therapy, recovery, and speech therapy can enable you to monitor your symptoms and carry on with an effective life.

Am I Going to Need a Wheelchair?

A great many people who have Multiple Sclerosis generally get around without assistance. However, there might be the point at which you'll have to utilize a cane or a walker to make it simpler. About 25% of individuals with the condition inevitably need a wheelchair.

Which Multiple Sclerosis Treatment Is Best for Me?

It's anything but difficult to feel overpowered by all the diverse drugs and treatments that can help individuals with Multiple Sclerosis.

The initial step is to find out about your treatment choices and discuss about them with your specialist. Consider how well the treatment should function, any conceivable reactions, how you'll take the treatment, and how it fits with your way of life.

Your doctor is a decent hotspot for data about the distinctive sorts of medications. He additionally can prescribe Multiple

Sclerosis support groups and different experts who can support you.

How Does Deep Brain Stimulation Help?

The fundamental objective of deep mind stimulation for Multiple Sclerosis is to ease shaking you can't control. It won't help with different issues, for example, loss of vision, feeling, or strength.

What Else Can Help Me?

An uplifting temperament can bring down your pressure and help you feel much improved.

Exercise procedures like jujitsu and yoga can loosen up you and give you more energy, balance, and adaptability. Continuously check with your specialist before you begin another fitness schedule. Try not to practice so hard that you feel depleted.

It's dependably a smart idea to eat a solid, all-around balanced diet as well. Ask your specialist what foods are directly for you.

What Is Optic Neuritis?

It's the inflammation of the nerve that links your eye to your brain. It can cause:

- Pain in the eye
- Blurred vision
- Graying of vision
- Blindness in one eye

In the event that you see any of these side effects, tell your specialist immediately. The way to protecting your eyesight is to get the issue early. Your doctor can treat you with steroids to battle the inflammation in the nerve.

Optic neuritis generally happens in one eye at once. However, it can influence both. It's regularly the primary indication that somebody has Multiple Sclerosis. About half of individuals with the condition will have optic neuritis in any event once.

In any case, it can happen to individuals who have other medical issues, as well, so it doesn't consequently imply that somebody has or will get Multiple Sclerosis.

A great many people with optic neuritis recovers completely, now and then with no treatment.

Keep up with Author Devon Goods, the Founder of Beyond My Diagnosis LLC, and publisher of:

- Multiple Sclerosis; All You Need to Know and Vital Solutions

- Beyond My Diagnosis; Steps to Coping with Sudden Illness

Want more? Visit: payhip.com/bmdsupport for

- Healthy Habit Tracker
- Beyond Planning 2019 Calendar
- Exercise and a Healthy Lifestyle
- Health and Fitness
- The Ultimate Exercise and Fitness Guide for Beginners

Join the Support Group via Facebook: bit.ly/bmdsupport

www.ingramcontent.com/pod-product-compliance
Lightning Source LLC
Chambersburg PA
CBHW051403280526
45784CB00007B/3083